BEYOND

60'S

"A Guide to Caring and Safeguarding the Elderly Around Us".

LINDA NWOSU, RN

TABLE OF CONTENTS

The Impact of Positive Relationships on the Elderly

Looking Forward to the Future of Elderly Care

CONCLUSION

INTRODUCTION

As the world population ages, it becomes increasingly paramount to care for and safeguard the elderly amongst us whether as a caregiver, family, friend or just someone interested in the welfare of the elderly. Beyond 60's is a special developmental stage in every individual's life and can be defined as a period of decline in physiological and cellular functions. It comes with a lot of changes and challenges which are considered a blessing by some and suffering by others, but at this phase of life, who suffers the most? The individual or the people around them?. I have heard several people say, 'I really can't imagine getting old and frail and depending on someone to care for me' This book would not only focus on how to care and safeguard the elderly but would also dedicate a chapter to certain options for the caregivers who are at a risk of a burnout.

However, despite the need to be free from the burden of caring for the aged and the struggles associated with it, have you ever wondered why this group of people are so significant in our lives and communities?. Sometimes, we feel they are too old and should be segregated from the society or that they have lived their lives and should make way for the younger generation but then, we can't do without them in every society.

First and foremost, despite the advanced age, they remain one of the most vulnerable groups in the society as a result of their declining age, social isolation and financial challenges. Thus, the importance of adequate care and support from people around them. In addition to this, they have contributed immensely to their families, communities and societies at large, so, the need to be appreciated by us. With regards to their life experiences, spending time with the elderly is a good way to learn and build a solid path for the future for the younger generation through making modifications from their life stories. Overall, caring and safeguarding the elderly is an effective way of ensuring that all individuals are able to live with dignity and respect as they age. Through my years of interacting with the elderly, I have learnt patience and empathy, therefore, being around them is a way of learning some core values, what about you?. As a young person, what is your attitude towards the beyond 60's whether family or not?. This book intends to serve as a guide towards caring and safeguarding the elderly as they approach the end of life while giving them the opportunity to enjoy this golden years.

The older adults also face various difficulties with regards to their age ranging from neglect, physical, emotional, financial, as well as medical challenges. Asides this, with technological advancements, these senior citizens also need to be educated on assistive technologies for independent living and the appropriate use of social media and online communities to build social networks, express their feelings without judgement and share their wisdom and experiences with others without being at risk of online bullying and harassment. Also, taking care of the elderly can be quite a challenging task, thus, it is important that caregivers adopt the resources available for them as indicated in this book. So I hope this book, 'Beyond 60's: A Guide to Caring and Safeguarding the Elderly Around Us' makes you understand the concepts of aging as it explores the unique needs of this age group, some of their challenges and gives you a practical guidance on how to help and protect the elderly in your lives while navigating health care, healthy living, financial planning and a supportive environment for them.

CHAPTER 1

UNDERSTANDING AGING

Imagine being born, enjoying the whole attention as a baby from people around you, tending to all your needs and taking proper care of you, then gradually with each passing year comes your birthday and you keep adding one year to your previous years. You grow from being a child to an adolescence to a young adult who takes up all the responsibilities, progressively you keep growing until you are beyond 60's, old and grey and depending on others to care for you once more just as when you were a neonate. That is my little explanation of aging and its processes and I hope you enjoy every bit of it when the time comes and help others around you who are already in this stage of life. Let's quickly look at how this changes occur known as the *Biology of aging*

Biology of Aging

This is a field of study that seeks to understand the underlying mechanisms of aging and how these changes occur. During the aging process, the body undergoes changes which affects the physical, psychological and emotional well-being.

There are different theories of aging which includes; the telomere theory, mitochondrial, and hormesis theory.

The telomere theory suggests that one of the major contributors of aging is the reduction in length of the telomeres which are the protective caps on the ends of our chromosomes. As these structures shorten over time, the cells ability to divide and regenerate reduces resulting in diverse age-related illnesses and conditions. The mitochondrial theory proposes that aging is related to an energy production decline in the power house of the cells while the hormesis theory states that being exposed to high levels of stress can be detrimental to health and longevity.

Another significant factor in aging is oxidative stress. This occurs when the body produces free radicals excessively which are unstable molecules, eventually damaging cells and leading to the development of chronic diseases like cancer, cardiovascular disease and neurodegenerative disorders.

Regardless of the numerous theories of aging, researchers concur that a combination of genetic, lifestyle and environmental factors play a part in the process of aging. Some of the major environmental factors include inadequate nutrition, lack of exercise and exposure to harmful substances such as cigarette smoking and air pollution. Despite the many advances in our comprehension of aging, there is still more to be learned about this multifaceted and complex process. We can develop new strategies for healthy aging promotion and prevention age-related ailments, helping us to enjoy longer healthier lives through our continuous exploration on the underlying mechanisms of aging,

Common Health Issues in Old Age

With old age, comes various health difficulties both physical and psychological issues due to the natural aging process and other factors. By understanding these common issues and management, we can help to improve the life of our elderly loved ones. Regular check-ups with a health care provider, a balanced diet, regular exercise and a healthy lifestyle can contribute to the prevention and management of these health issues and help the elderly to enjoy a prolonged and more satisfying life. Some common health issues amongst others include:

Cardiovascular Disease

Cardiovascular disease refers to conditions that affect the heart and blood vessels, including high blood pressure, heart disease, and stroke. Risk factors for cardiovascular disease include a sedentary lifestyle, smoking, high blood pressure, and high cholesterol levels. Treatment for cardiovascular disease may include medication, lifestyle changes, and surgery in severe cases.

Dementia

Dementia is a group of conditions that affect the brain, leading to a decline in cognitive abilities. It can cause memory loss, confusion, and difficulty with daily tasks. There are various types of dementia, including Alzheimer's disease, vascular dementia, and Lewy body dementia. Although there is no cure for dementia, medication and therapy can help manage symptoms and improve quality of life.

Osteoporosis

Osteoporosis is a bone disease that causes bones to become weak and brittle, leading to a higher risk of fractures. It is caused by a loss of bone density, which is more common in women after menopause. Treatment for osteoporosis may include medication, a balanced diet rich in calcium and vitamin D, and exercise to improve bone strength.

Diabetes

Diabetes is a chronic condition that affects the body's ability to produce or use insulin, leading to high blood sugar levels. It can cause a range of complications, including nerve damage, kidney damage, and eye problems. Treatment for diabetes may include medication, dietary changes, and regular monitoring of blood sugar levels.

Arthritis

Arthritis is a joint disease that affects millions of people worldwide, particularly the elderly. It is caused by the wear and tear of cartilage in the joints, leading to pain, stiffness, and swelling. Treatment for arthritis may include pain management, exercise, and medication to slow down the progression of the disease.

Depression

Depression is a mental health condition that can affect people of all ages, including the elderly. It can cause feelings of sadness, hopelessness, and loss of interest in daily activities. Treatment for depression may include therapy, medication, and lifestyle changes

The World Health Organization mentions that one of the characteristics of older age is the emergence of several complex health states known as geriatric syndromes which results from multiple underlying factors and include urinary continence, falls, pressure sores, and delirium. Other health changes in the elderly include back and neck pain, hearing loss, respiratory diseases as well as refractive errors and vision loss.

The Impact of Social and Environmental Factors

Aging is a natural process that affects everyone. However, the rate and experience of aging can vary greatly among individuals. Research has shown that social and environmental factors in their homes, neighborhoods and communities can significantly impact the aging process. These factors can affect health directly or through barriers that affect decisions, opportunities and health behavior, and with a friendly environment, these individuals would be able to cope despite their incapability. A supportive environment is one that put their needs into consideration such as the provision of safe and accessible buildings which are easy to navigate, and transport facilities.

Social Factors

Social factors such as social support, social engagement, and social isolation have been linked to the aging process. Social support, which includes emotional, informational, and tangible support from others, has been found to improve physical and mental health, reduce stress, and increase longevity. Social engagement, which involves participating in social activities such as volunteering, attending social events, and joining clubs or groups, has also been linked to better physical and mental health in older adults. In contrast, social isolation has been associated with negative health outcomes, including increased risk of depression, cognitive decline, and mortality.

Environmental Factors

Environmental factors such as air pollution, access to green spaces, and neighborhood walkability have also been linked to the aging process. Air pollution has been shown to increase the risk of cardiovascular and respiratory diseases, which can accelerate the aging process. On the other hand, access to green spaces such as parks and forests has been associated with better physical and mental health in older adults. Similarly, living in neighborhoods with good walkability, which includes factors such as sidewalks, streetlights, and traffic safety, has been linked to better physical health and mobility in older adults.

In conclusion, social and environmental factors can have a significant impact on the aging process. Social support, social engagement, access to green spaces, and neighborhood walkability can improve physical and mental health in older adults, while social isolation and air pollution can have negative health outcomes. Understanding the impact of these factors on aging can help individuals, communities, and policymakers take steps to promote healthy aging and improve the quality of life for older adults.

CHAPTER 2

CARING FOR THE ELDERLY

This chapter provides adequate guidance to taking care of the aged. Their hygiene, dietary habits, exercise and mobility as well as emotional support and how to communicate effectively with them. To be honest, as a health care worker, I have gotten to realize that the elderly can be a difficult group to work with. The mode of communication matters to them and it requires being done in a unique way which would still maintain that dignity and respect. Most times, they act as children so while being firm with regards to some of their decisions, you also have to be loving. A detailed personal experience was a situation where an elderly woman in her 80's who was hospitalized wanted to be discharged to travel to her hometown to check on her farm land, regardless of the pleas from her children on the need to stay, all proved abortive. But you know what, knowing how to go around communicating with the elderly, I made her stay until she was fully recovered to the surprise of her children, and they left the health facility with smiles on their faces. I will be teaching you the same tactics through this chapter.

Providing Physical Care: Hygiene, Nutrition and Mobility

Hygiene

Maintaining a good personal hygiene is very essential across all ages and helps to reduce the incidence of diseases. It entails proper grooming and care from the head to toe of an individual. For the new born as well as the elderly, their hygiene and its maintenance is mostly dependent on the carers and the people around them. In most cases, attending to this need of theirs can be a herculean task just like a friend of mine, Sarah once told me, ' I really don't know how to handle granny's hygiene. It has become a torn in my flesh. She literally messes up the whole room. She bed wets and soils herself, yet, she can't clean herself up. I am really tired and caring for her is really draining me'

In an elderly person, there can actually be a case of urinary and fecal continence. They can't hold it in even if they want to. So, just like I told Sarah on how to handle this situation, I would be sharing some tips which would go a long way for you and helps to ensure that you still maintain that healthy relationship with them without any strain due to hygiene shortcomings.

Firstly, you have to accept that this people are aged and would need all the care they can get. Most times, they want to be independent and still be that strong person they have always been but age and time is not on their side. Get a carer or someone to help you run shifts in taking care of your aged loved ones, get quality adult diapers and change immediately when soiled to ensure their comfort. Reassure them that it is something you can handle and that they are not a burden so that their psychological health will be intact.

Nutrition

The best food at this stage of life are natural foods and foods that contain essential nutrients like protein such as meat, fish, and eggs, calcium, iron and vitamins that will boosts their body repair, bone growth, anti-oxidants production, and reduce the incidence of certain diseases like hypertension and diabetes. At this stage, do not be surprised when they consume less food and are filled quickly. Sometimes, they can be quite picky with foods, there can be a change of diet from solid foods to puree diets.

Growing up and watching my mum feed my grand dad, I always wondered why she would always shred the meats while serving him as they were his favorite food. As an adult, I think I have my answer, my grand dad didn't have much teeth left in his mouth to chew some tough foods, a difficulty most of them experience.

So, regardless of the situation, find alternatives towards making them enjoy every bit of their meal as much as they can consume and prevent malnutrition. Draft a healthy meal plan with the help of a dietician/nutritionist and give them a satisfying nutritional experience.

Some of the best foods at this stage includes; fruits and vegetables, high fiber diets and water which would help in the prevention of constipation which is a common challenge in the elderly.

According to Alice Callahan , the older population requires less calories than the younger adults due to a decline in lean body mass and metabolic rate. For women in this age range, the energy requirement is between 1600 and 2,200 calories while that of men is between 2000 and 2800, depending on the activity level. Dietary choices can address some of the nutritional challenges at this stage and can improve their health and well-being, therefore, it is an essential part to consider.

Mobility

Physical activity is reduced in the elderly and due to bone loss that comes with aging, so many of them have difficulties in walking and engaging in activities of daily living. These limitations can cause serious health effects such as formation of thrombus which can lodge in the heart or brain causing heart diseases and stroke.

For the aged ones who can still walk around on their own, how do I really get to help them? Below are tips to assist the mobile aged ones around you.

- Appropriate lighting in the environment would definitely help to reduce the risks of falls.
- Application of bed rails to prevent falls or putting their mattress on a lower level to reduce the height which would be safer for them.
- Provision of urinals or bed pan closer to them especially during the night time to reduce that walking distance.

- Keeping the environment clean and free from water spillages and even substances that can cause falls like banana peels.
- Provision of assistive walking devices like canes, walkers and crutches.

For the bedridden ones, their condition doesn't stop them from exercising, as much as you can, assist them in range of motion exercises; try to move their joints regularly in order to prevent muscle wastage and bone stiffness.

Providing Emotional Support

As people age, they may encounter diverse physical, emotional and social changes that can impact their overall well-being. Although physical health may be the most obvious change, it is also important to address the emotional needs of the elderly. Emotional support can provide a sense of comfort and security to the elderly, which can have a positive impact on their psychological and physical health. This guide aims to provide caregivers with tips and strategies for providing adequate emotional support to the elderly. It will explore the common emotional difficulties faced by the older adults and offer practical advice on how to address them. Due to the social isolation towards the elderly, health problems or loss of a loved one, they tend to face a variety of emotional challenges such as withdrawal, loneliness, anxiety, fear and depression which affects their mental health. At this advanced age, there are certain conditions which has severe effects on the elderly such as dementia. So, it is paramount to recognize and address these emotions to provide the best possible emotional support.

Tips for providing emotional support

- Listening: One of the most essential thins you can do to provide emotional support is to listen to the elderly. Give them a chance to express their feelings and be an active listener. Make eye contact while they talk and show that you are genuinely interested in what they are saying. Sometimes, all they need is someone who is willing to listen to them

- Spend time with them: Spending time with the aged ones helps to alleviate feelings of isolation and loneliness. Plan activities that they enjoy and participate in it with them. It can be something as simple as playing a game, talking a walk or even watching a genre of movie they love together.

- Encourage social interaction: This is critical to emotional well-being. They should be included in social activities and encouraged to participate effectively. This helps to reduce the feelings of loneliness and promotes a sense of community.

- Show empathy: Empathy means putting yourself in someone else's shoes and understanding their perspective which is an essential component of emotional support. Validate their feelings and let them know that you understand and care.

- Provide physical comfort: Offering a warm blanket or a gentle touch, shows love and can provide a sense of security and comfort to the elderly. If appropriate, offer hugs and physical contact to show that you care.

Conclusively, providing emotional support to the elderly is important to their overall well-being. By understanding their emotional needs and utilizing this tips and strategies provided in this guide, caregivers an make a remarkable difference in the lives of the elderly.

Communicating Effectively with the Elderly

The elderly can sometimes be one of the most difficult people to communicate with. Maybe, because they feel they are older and can independently make decisions for themselves or they feel they can't be taking orders or instructions from the younger ones around them or it can be due to physical and cognitive changes that affect their ability to communicate effectively. Effective communication with this age group requires patience, attentiveness and empathy. By being mindful of their special needs and challenges, you can improve the understanding and connection, leading to a more fulfilling and enjoying communication between both parties. Thus, if you have been having difficulties communicating with an elderly person, then this is for you as we explore ways for an effective communication taking into consideration their unique needs and challenges.

1. Speak clearly and slowly: The elderly may have difficulties in hearing or understanding speech, so it is essential to speak slowly and clearly. Avoid the use of complex words or long sentence that could confuse them. Face them when speaking. And maintain eye contact to show that you are listening actively.

2. Be patient and attentive: Give the elderly enough time to process what you are saying before expecting a feedback as they may take longer to process information and respond, so it is essential

to be patient and attentive. Avoid interrupting or finishing their sentences as this can be frustrating to them and may make them feel dismissed.

3. Be mindful of Non-verbal communication: Nonverbal cues such as body language and facial expressions can be misinterpreted by the elderly. Therefore, it is crucial to be mindful of your body languages and facial expressions, ensuring that they match what you are saying.

4. Use of positive languages: This can improve the communication experience of both parties. Instead of focusing on their limitations, focus on what they can do. For example, rather than saying, ''You can't do that, '' say, ''Let's find another way to get that done''. Positive language can help them feel valued and respected.

5. Use memory aids: Memory aids such as calendars or notes can help the elderly keep track of important information such as appointments or

medication schedules as they can be forgetful. Visual aids such as pictures or diagrams can also help them understand complex information.

6. Show empathy and compassion: The elderly may face several challenges, including loneliness, illness, or loss of independence. It is vital to show empathy and compassion when communicating with them. Listen to their concerns, acknowledge their feelings rather than arguing with them or putting their emotions aside and offer support and reassurance.

CHAPTER 3

ELDER ABUSE AND NEGLECT

Elder abuse and neglect can be defined as any action or lack of action that causes harm and distress to an older person and this is a serious issue affecting many older adults across the globe. This can include physical, sexual, or emotional abuse, as well as financial exploitation or neglect. Elder abuse can occur in various places including, the individual's home, a nursing home, a friend's place or even an assisted living place and can be initiated by either the caregivers, relatives, health care providers, strangers or friends. It is quite unfortunate that most cases of elder abuse go unnoticed for a long period of time and are underreported, leaving the elderly vulnerable to further maltreatment.

Physical abuse can include hitting, pushing or restraining an older person. Even though some elderly persons may be forgetful and may want to leave or go outside the house on their own, it doesn't give the caregiver the right to lock him/her up. Find a better means to ensure their safety while respecting their freedom of movement. Emotional abuse can include threats, verbal abuse, ignoring the older adult or isolation from family and friends. Sexual abuse entails any unwanted sexual advances or contact or forcing an older person to watch sexual acts. Financial exploitation can include stealing money or property, forging signatures, pressuring an older person into giving away their assets. Neglect can include failing to provide adequate food, clothing and medical care. Every elderly person is entitled to appropriate care and provision of basic life needs from people around them.

There are several factors contributing to the increase in elder abuse and neglect. These include mental or physical illness, social isolation, cognitive impairment and a lack of caregiver training or support. In addition, older adults who are members of a marginalized society are at a higher risk of abuse and neglect due to factors such as discrimination, poverty and lack of resources.

Prevention of elder abuse and neglect requires a community effort and it is important to note that the abuse and neglect is not the fault of the older person and it is unacceptable. This can be mitigated by education and awareness on elder abuse and neglect which can help to reduce the stigma surrounding the issue and increase the reporting of abuse and neglect and being vigilant for signs of abuse and reporting to appropriate authorities such as adult protective services, law enforcement, or to a health care provider.

Types of Elder Abuse and Neglect

As already discussed above, there five major types of elder abuse and neglect and they include:

- Physical abuse
- Sexual abuse
- Emotional abuse
- Financial abuse
- Neglect

Warning Signs

Kenneth's Story

'Kenneth, a young man in his 30's had a friend in his neighborhood named Jeffrey, an 83 year old man who he loves spending the weekend with. On several occasions, he noticed some bruises on Jeffrey's body but thought it was a result of falls. Until one faithful day, unknown to the caregiver, he walked into the living room only to see Jeffrey tied to a chair and being flogged by the caregiver because he soiled his clothes. Kenneth quickly stopped that unbearable sight from further occurring and called the authorities. Jeffrey was not being hurt only physically but was traumatized'.

If only Kenneth was more vigilant and knew the warning signs of elder abuse and neglect, he would have acted earlier. The warning signs include

- Withdrawal from activities they enjoy doing.
- Having troubles sleeping.

- Looks unkempt from head to toe.

- Acts agitated or violent.

- Displays signs of trauma.

- Has unexplained bruises and cuts

- Significant weight loss without any reason

- Lacks medical aids such as walkers, glasses or hearing aids

- Has pressure sores and other preventable conditions.

- Shows signs of insufficient care and unpaid bills despite abundant financial resources.

- Stays in unsafe and hazardous living conditions.

How to Report Abuse and Neglect

Once you notice a sign of abuse, try to ask further questions on what is going on when you are alone with the elderly person because the abuser can be anyone around them. Although, they might be in fear or try to protect the abuser due to the relationship they have with them or feel ashamed to report the mistreatment, step in and help. Let them know that you can be of help and they can equally receive help if they speak out. With or without prove, report what you see to adult protective services and they will definitely take it up from there or if the elderly person is living in a long-term care facility, such as a nursing home, you can also contact the state agency responsible for licensing and regulating these facilities. This may be a department of health or a department of social services. They can investigate and take action against the facility if necessary. If you suspect financial abuse or exploitation, you can contact your local law enforcement agency or your state attorney general's office. They may be able to investigate and prosecute those responsible for the abuse or exploitation

When reporting abuse or neglect of an elderly person, it is important to provide as much information as possible, including the name and address of the elderly person, the nature of the abuse or neglect, the name of the alleged abuser, and any other relevant details. Remember, it is better to report suspected abuse and neglect than to remain silent and allow it to continue.

CHAPTER 4

LEGAL AND FINANCIAL ISSUES

The elderly are usually prone to financial exploitations and neglect. A situation where the people around them want to forcefully take over what they have worked for over the years or the misuse and mismanagement of their assets. In cases of neglect, the financial responsibilities of the elderly are not being cared for. Their social, economic, physical and medical needs that money can solve are not being attended to.

The beyond 60's are always faced with the challenges of making their will, how to share their properties and assets and getting a trustworthy legal practitioner who would uphold and maintain their decisions and would not succumb to the pressures of relatives even after they are gone.

A friend of mine once shared a story with me of a particular wealthy family and what took place between the siblings and relatives after the breadwinner of the family, a man of 75 years was no more. Sometimes you may think it doesn't matter and your family is at peace, but not when assets and properties worth so much value are involved. The human heart can be deceptive at times, you know. So how was this issue resolved in that family?. Unknown to them, the man left a will with his lawyer which they found out later after it was disclosed to them and read in the presence of everyone. Imagine what would have happened if he didn't prepare this legal document before his death or if he didn't have a trustworthy lawyer?. In this chapter, we would be talking about wills and trusts, the power of attorney and how to prevent conflict over your will even after you are no more.

Wills and Trusts

These are legal documents which are powerful tools that can be used to protect the assets and interests of senior citizens who may be vulnerable to abuse and neglect. Wills and trusts are estate planning tools that can be used to provide for loved ones after a person's death. They can also be used to set aside assets for specific purposes, such as charitable giving or the care of a loved one with special needs. In cases of elder abuse or neglect, wills and trusts can be used to ensure that an elderly person's assets are protected and used for their intended purposes.

One important tool for protecting seniors is a will. A will is a legal document that specifies how a person's assets will be distributed after their death. This can be an important tool for preventing family members or caregivers from taking advantage of an elderly person after they pass away. By specifying how their assets will be distributed, a senior can ensure that their wishes are respected and that their assets are used for the intended purposes.

Another important tool that can be used to protect seniors from abuse and neglect is the revocable living trust. This type of trust is established during a person's lifetime and can be changed or revoked at any time. The trust assets are managed by a trustee, who is often the person creating the trust. In the case of elder abuse or neglect, a revocable living trust can provide a mechanism for an elderly person to maintain control of their assets while still having a trusted person manage those assets.

Power of Attorney

In addition to a revocable living trust, a durable power of attorney can be another important tool for seniors. A durable power of attorney is a legal document that appoints someone to act on behalf of an elderly person in the event they become unable to make decisions for themselves. This can be useful in situations where an elderly person is being abused or neglected and needs someone to step in and protect their interests.

Tips to Prevent Conflicts Over Your Will as an Elderly Even When You Are Gone

So if you have gotten to this chapter of this book, whether you are reading as an elderly person or a younger person, this would give you a guide on the best way to handle this legal and financial issues that may arise.

This requires proper planning and communication. By following the tips below, you would be able to learn how to handle these issues, protect your legacy and maintain harmony and peace within your family even in your absence.

1. Start with Communication: One of the best ways to prevent conflicts over your will is to communicate with your loved ones. Talk to your family members about your estate plans, including the distribution of assets and personal items. Explain your reasoning behind your decisions and listen to their concerns. By being transparent, you can avoid misunderstandings and resentment.

2. Hire a Professional: It's essential to work with an attorney who specializes in estate planning. They can help you navigate the legalities of creating a will and ensure your wishes are carried out. Additionally, they can help you make informed decisions about your assets and answer any questions you have about the process.

3. Update Your Will Regularly: As your circumstances change, it is essential to update your will to reflect your current situation. Whether it's a new marriage, divorce, or the birth of a grandchild, keeping your will up to date ensures that your wishes are always updated. This would help to prevent misunderstandings and disputes.

4. Consider a Trust: Creating a trust is an excellent way to ensure your assets are distributed according to your wishes. By establishing a trust, you can avoid probate, which can be a lengthy and expensive process. Additionally, you can name a trustee who will oversee the distribution of assets, which can prevent disputes over personal items and property.

5. Keep Personal Items Separate: Personal items can hold significant emotional value to family members. To prevent conflicts, consider designating specific items to certain people in your will. However, it's essential to keep personal

items separate from other assets, as they can't be divided equally. By being clear and transparent about who receives which item, you can avoid disagreements.

Overall, planning for these golden years in terms of finances is very essential. As a older person, it is important to correct the misconception that your children are a ticket to your old age and even as a younger person, do not put that burden on your children. Sure, children can be your insurance but remember, you also have to find a means to lighten their burdens as they would be having other responsibilities. Plan towards these and I am certain that you will enjoy these stage of life while adopting the necessary legal measures.

CHAPTER 5

RESOURCES FOR CAREGIVERS

A caregiver is someone who provides care, support, and assistance to individuals who are unable to care for themselves due to age, illness, disability, or other limitations. Caregivers can be family members, friends, or professionals, and they may provide physical, emotional, or financial support to their care recipients. The responsibilities of a caregiver can vary widely depending on the needs of the person they are caring for, and may include tasks such as bathing, feeding, administering medication, providing transportation, managing finances, and providing companionship and emotional support.

Caregiving can be a challenging, difficult and demanding but rewarding role, and requires a great deal of compassion, patience, and dedication. If you are experiencing this, know that you are not alone in this journey. Sometimes, you have to shuffle between taking care of their physical needs, taking them for their medical check up and even catering to their financial needs which can really be demanding on your personal life. In certain situations, you have to leave a paying job and inconvenience yourself just to take up this new responsibilities. It can even be harder when there is no improvement on their physical and mental health.

However, despite your will to take care of them effectively, you ought to take care of yourself and your needs first, so that you can give in the best you can while providing care for them. There are certain support groups and respite care which can be of help and give you a break as a caregiver based on arrangements.

Support Groups

There are various support groups for caregivers and the choice is dependent on you, the caregiver. These groups provide a safe and supportive environment where caregivers can share their experiences, express their feelings without judgement, receive emotional support and gain useful information and resources. Support groups can be organized in different ways, either in-person meetings which provides the opportunities for caregivers to interact face-to-face and build a sense of community, virtual meetings which can be beneficial for those who live in rural areas or have mobility issues or online forums where caregivers can be anonymous and freely express themselves through writing. Some of the support groups include:

1. Caregiver-specific support groups: Many organizations, such as the Alzheimer's Association, offer caregiver-specific support groups. These groups provide a safe and supportive environment for caregivers to share their experiences, ask questions, and offer advice to one another. Some groups may be specific to caregivers of individuals with certain conditions, such as dementia or Parkinson's disease.

2. Online support groups: For caregivers who may not be able to attend in-person support groups, online support groups can be a great option. These groups can be found on social media platforms or

on websites dedicated to caregiving. They offer a virtual community where caregivers can share their experiences and offer support to one another.

3. Support groups for specific demographics: Some support groups are specifically geared towards certain demographic groups, such as men or LGBT+ caregivers. These groups may offer a more specialized focus on issues that are unique to those demographics, such as the challenges of caregiving as a same-sex couple.

4. Faith-based support groups: For caregivers who find comfort in their faith, faith-based support groups can offer a unique type of support. These groups may be held at local churches or other places of worship and provide a supportive environment for caregivers to connect with others who share their beliefs.

5. Caregiver coaching: Some organizations offer caregiver coaching to help caregivers navigate

their care giving role. This can include one-on-one coaching sessions or group coaching sessions, where caregivers can learn new skills and strategies for managing their care giving responsibilities.

Respite Care

Respite care is a service designed to provide temporary relief to family caregivers who are caring for elderly or disabled loved ones. This can help reduce the stress and burden of caregiving and give caregivers the opportunity to rest, take care of their own needs, and engage in other activities that they enjoy. Respite care can be beneficial for both the caregiver and the senior, including improved mental health and reduced stress for the caregiver, and socialization and engagement for the senior. It can also help prevent caregiver burnout and reduce the risk of elder abuse or neglect. Respite care can take many forms, including:

- In-home respite care: A professional caregiver comes to the home and provides care for the senior, allowing the family caregiver to take a break.

- Adult day care: The senior attends a program at a center during the day, where they receive care and participate in activities, while the family caregiver takes a break.

- Residential respite care: The senior stays at a residential care facility for a short period, while the family caregiver takes a break.

- Respite vacations: The caregiver and their loved one can go on vacation together, with the assistance of a professional caregiver.

Assisted Living Options

Assisted living is an option for caregivers of elderly individuals who may require additional support and services to maintain their quality of life. Assisted living communities offer a range of services including assistance with daily activities, healthcare services, medication management, social and recreational activities, and transportation.

When considering assisted living options, it's important to keep in mind the individual needs and preferences of the elderly person being cared for. Some things to consider when looking for an assisted living community include:

- Location: Is the community located in a safe and accessible area that is convenient for family and friends to visit?

- Services and amenities: What types of services and amenities are offered, such as meals, housekeeping, laundry, transportation, and social activities? Are there additional fees for these services?

- Staff qualifications: What are the qualifications of the staff who will be providing care? Are they trained to provide specialized care for individuals with specific health conditions?

- Cost: What is the cost of living in the community, and what services are included in that cost? Is financial assistance available for those who need it?

- Resident and family satisfaction: What do current and former residents and their families have to say about their experience with the community?

It's also important to take a tour of any potential assisted living communities to get a sense of the atmosphere, cleanliness and overall feel of the community. Talking to current residents and staff can also provide valuable insights into the quality of care provided.

Assisted living can be a beneficial option for caregivers of the elderly, providing a supportive and safe environment for their loved one while also allowing the caregiver to take a step back and prioritize their own self-care.

CHAPTER 6

TECHNOLOGY FOR THE ELDERLY

Technology has the power to revolutionize the lives of people of all ages, including the elderly. With the growing technological advancement, it is essential that the elderly are taught how to use the media, the benefits it can bring to them for instance, joining online communities where they can share their worries, life situations and also learn certain ways to handle them, managing their health challenges, building social connections and living independently. Appropriate teaching on the use of technological devices helps them to be more independent and protects them from abuse, neglect, online bullying and harassment. This chapter focuses on ways technology can be beneficial to seniors and the importance of carers using this tool to care and safeguard the elderly.

Assistive Technology for Independent Living

There are various technological devices that can assist seniors to perform various tasks ranging from communication, mobility, medication management and personal safety and to live an independent life. Such devices include smartphone, tablets, computers, hearing aids and wearable technology which can have several features for easier use like large buttons, voice commands and easy-to-use interface.

In cases of home automation and safety, smart home devices such as voice-activated assistants like google assistant or Amazon's Alexa , automated lighting and temperature control, home security devices can be of great benefits to the elderly. Installing stair lifts can help them walk up and down the stairs with ease, smart locks gives them the control to allow specific people into their homes, grab bars can help them maintain balance and prevent falls in the bathroom and personal emergency response systems can be introduced which can be worn in form of a necklace or bracelet and can be activated with the touch of a button in cases of emergency. There are numerous of this devices, therefore, it is essential that the assistive devices chosen are appropriate with the needs of the elderly.

Telehealth and Telemedicine

Technology can be used to promote better health and wellness for the elderly in the form of telehealth and telemedicine, fitness trackers and medication management tools. Telehealth and telemedicine provides patients with health care services and allows healthcare providers to offer medical care from a distance. It refers to the use of technology to provide healthcare remotely. Although 'telehealth' and 'telemedicine' are used interchangeably, there is a subtle difference between them.

Telehealth refers to a broader range of services and encompasses telemedicine. It includes not only clinical services but also non-clinical services such as health education, health promotion and administrative activities and can be defined as the delivery of healthcare services and information through telecommunications technologies, such as videoconferencing, remote monitoring, and mobile health apps. On the other hand, telemedicine focuses primarily on the provision of clinical services including consultation, diagnosis and treatment.

Although these technologies have various challenges such as the need for reliable internet connectivity and access to technology, data and privacy issues, and lack of personal interaction, it offers great benefits, which includes increased access to healthcare services, reduced health care cost, convenience and improved patient outcomes.

There are different types of telehealth and telemedicine service and they include:

- Virtual Consultations: These are consultations with doctors or other healthcare providers that take place over video or phone calls or chat platforms. Patients can discuss their symptoms, receive diagnoses, and get prescriptions without leaving their homes.

- Remote Monitoring: Remote monitoring involves using devices to collect data about patients' health and share it with healthcare providers. This can include things like heart rate monitors, blood glucose monitors, and other types of wearable technology. Remote monitoring can be particularly useful for aged people with chronic conditions, as it allows healthcare workers to monitor their health status and adjust treatment plans as required.

- Electronic Health Records: Electronic health records allow healthcare providers to access patients' medical histories and other important information remotely. This can improve communication between different providers and help ensure that patients receive the best possible care.

- Health Education: Telehealth and telemedicine can also be used to provide health education to patients. This can include virtual classes or resources that patients can access from home.

Overall, it is essential that people around the elderly adopt these new technological developments to improve the quality of care given to the elderly and gives them the opportunity to focus on other aspects of care.

Social Media and Online Communities

In recent times, social media and online communities have become a ubiquitous part of our daily lives and this is not just for young people but senior citizens can benefit from these platforms as well. Through these channels which technology has encouraged, older adults can build social connections and join online communities where they can make friends, learn a lot, share their wisdom and experiences gathered over the years and connect with the world. Whether you are a senior yourself reading this book or you are looking for ways to help the ones in your life, consider exploring some of the social media platforms and online communities available today. However, it is the duty of the carer to ensure that they are staying safe online and that their personal information is protected.

Types of social media and online communities for the elderly

There are numerous social media platforms and online communities that are specifically designed for older adults. Some of the popular options include:

1. Facebook: Facebook is one of the most popular social media platforms for people of all ages. Seniors can use it to connect with friends and family members, join groups related to their interests, and share photos and updates with others.

2. Nextdoor: Nextdoor is a social media platform that connects people who live in the same neighborhood. This can be a great way for seniors to stay connected with their local community, get updates on local events, and even find help from neighbors if they need it.

3. AARP Community: The AARP (American Association of Retired Persons) Community is an online forum where seniors can connect with

others from around the country. The forum covers a wide range of topics, from health and wellness to travel and entertainment.

4. Silver Surfers: Silver Surfers is an online community that is specifically designed for seniors. It offers a wide range of resources, including forums, news articles, and expert advice on topics that are relevant to seniors.

CHAPTER 7
VALUE OF CARING FOR THE ELDERLY

Sometimes, you wonder what the value of caring for the elderly is. Value refers to the degree of importance given to something. Thus, it includes giving attention and love to this age group so that they can live a long life free from anxiety and worries. Although caring for them can be challenging, it can also be rewarding for both the caregiver and the older adult.

The Impact of Positive Relationships on the Elderly

Spending time with the elderly, I have come to realize that they cherish quality time and are always over the moon when a loved one or friend spends time with them. This made me realize that positive relationships has a great impact on the elderly. It improves their general health and well-being and as society ages, it is important to recognize the value of positive relationships in promoting the health and happiness of older adults and to provide resources and support to promote such relationships. Nevertheless, asides putting smiles on their faces, there are other significance it has on them and these positive relationships can be in various ways.

Social Support

Social support is the assistance or care provided by others, such as family members, friends, or community members. It is a key factor in promoting the well-being of older adults. Research has shown that older adults with strong social support systems have better physical and mental health, lower rates of depression and anxiety, and higher life satisfaction.

Social Activities

Social activities can also provide older adults with opportunities to engage in meaningful and enjoyable experiences, leading to a sense of purpose and connection. Participating in group activities, such as book clubs, exercise classes, or religious groups, can help older adults maintain their social connections and prevent feelings of loneliness.

Intergenerational Relationships

Intergenerational relationships, or connections between people of different age groups, can also be beneficial for older adults. Such relationships can provide opportunities for learning, sharing wisdom, and enjoying the company of younger people. Additionally, intergenerational relationships can help older adults feel more connected to their communities and reduce feelings of social isolation.

Caregiving Relationships

Caregiving relationships, in which an older adult receives assistance and care from a family member or friend, can also be beneficial. Caregivers can provide emotional support, practical help, and companionship.

Looking Forward to the Future of Elderly Care.
Over the past few decades, the field of elderly care has seen significant advancements, and the future looks bright as we continue to push the boundaries of what is possible. With the increasing aging population, in the forthcoming

years, a lot of changes would occur with the environment and health care in consideration of senior citizens. The environment would be more friendly and appropriate with their needs. Also, with advancement in technology such as advances in robotics, AI and wearables, the older adults are already experiencing a greater impact in their lives and as these technologies continue to improve, we anticipate to see more innovative solutions for elderly care. In the future, the health care system would provide more quality services. In most countries presently, there is a shift in the mode of delivery of elderly care. Many countries are moving away from traditional care models, such as nursing homes, and are instead focusing on community-based care. This approach allows elderly people to receive care in their own homes or within their local community, enabling them to maintain their independence and social connections. It also has the potential to reduce costs associated with elderly care and decrease the burden on hospitals. Individuals are getting more enlightened on the need to care effectively for the elderly and show greater concerns towards how to ameliorate the challenges they face.

Therefore, the future of elderly care is exciting, and there is much to be optimistic about. With the continued development of technology, the shift towards community-based care, and a greater focus on education and awareness of individuals on the needs of the aged amongst us, we can ensure that elderly people receive the care they deserve. As we move forward, let us continue to prioritize elderly care and work towards a brighter future for all

CONCLUSION

The Beyond 60's are an essential group in the society despite being frail due to their advanced age and the many health challenges they face. They are a group who we can learn from based on their overall life experiences. Thus, it is important that they are cared for and safeguarded from all forms of abuse and neglect.

In this book, we have explored various topics on aging, understanding how this process occurs, their various challenges including physical, emotional, and health challenges, the legal and financial issues they encounter, different types of elder abuse and neglect, how they can be managed, and resources available for the caregivers who are at risk of a burnout while caring for them. Interestingly, it also looked into technology for the elderly, the impact of positive relationships on the elderly and the future of elderly care.

Finally, if you are reading this book, 'Beyond 60's: A Guide to Caring and Safeguarding the Elderly Around Us' as an older adult or just simply someone who is interested in the care and welfare of the elderly, I hope it meets your needs in several aspects of their care.